FRUIT

HARMONY

SIPPERS

Enjoy A Symphony Of Harmonious Fruit Flavors.

5. HARMONIZED FRUITS 4: PINEAPPLE HEAVEN FUSION

- Preparation steps

- Ingredients

- Benefits

- Storage

6. HARMONIZED FRUITS 5: MELON MAGIC SYMPHONY

- Preparation steps

- Ingredients

- Benefits

- Storage

7. HARMONIZED FRUITS 6: TROPICAL BREEZES FUSION

- Preparation steps

- Ingredients

- Benefits

- Storage

8. HARMONIZED FRUITS 7: APPLEORCHARD SYMPHONY

- Preparation steps

- Ingredients

- Benefits

- Storage

9. HARMONIZED FRUITS 8: KIWI KALEIDOSCOPE REFRESHER

- Preparation steps

- Ingredients

- Benefits

- Storage

10. HARMONIZED FRUITS 9: SUNSET PEACH SOOTHER

- Preparation steps

- Ingredients

- Benefits

- Storage

11. HARMONIZED FRUITS 10: GUAVA GLOW ELIXIR

- Preparation steps

- Ingredients

- Benefits

- Storage

INTRODUCTION

Step into the mesmerizing realm of "Fruit Symphony Sippers: Immerse yourself in a Symphony of Melodious Flavors." Within the captivating pages of this spellbinding eBook, weextend an invitation to luxuriate in the delectable symphonies forged by the union of nature's most exquisite fruits. Every sip unveils a harmonious fusion of vibrant hues, tantalizing scents, and exquisite tastes, meticulously choreographed to bestow upon you a matchless and invigorating encounter. From the succulent crescendos of tropical fruits to the velvety ballads of berries, our recipes not only enthrall your senses but also saturate your being with the bounty of vitamins and antioxidants. Embark on this odyssey through a symphony of flavors, exalting the pureand succulent tastes that nature has so graciously bestowed upon us.

HARMONIZED FRUITS 1

MANGO TANGO SENSATION

Preparation:

1. Extract the pit from the ripe mangoes.

2. Shape the mango tissue into lumps.

3. Introduce the mango chunks intoa blender.

4. Blitz until velvety.

5. Alternatively, strain toeliminateany sinewy bits.

Ingredients:

- Ripe mangoes - Water (as required)

Benefits:

- Abounds in L-ascorbic acid and A - Possesses cancer-preventing attributes

- Facilitates absorption and augments resistance

- Elevates skin health

Storage:

Refrigerate in an airtight receptacle for a maximum of 3 days. Vigorously shake before serving.

HARMONIZED FRUITS 2

BERRY IMPACT MEDLEY

Preparation:

1. Purify and cleanse the strawberries, blueberries, and raspberries.

2. Integrate the berries intoa blender

3. Blitz until smooth.

Ingredients:

- Strawberries - Blueberries - Raspberries - Water (optional)

Benefits:

- Rich in anti-cancer agents

- Fosters heart well-being

- Amplifies brain capacity

- Enhances skin vitality

Storage:

Refrigerate in an airtight receptacle for a maximum of 2 days. Vigorously shake before serving.

HARMONIZED FRUITS 3

CITRUS SONG ELIXIR

Preparation:

1. Remove the peels and quarter theoranges and grapefruits.

2. Extract juice from the lemons by pressing them.

3. Combine the citrus segments and lemon juice in a blender.

4. Blitz until smooth.

Ingredients:

- Oranges - Grapefruit - Lemons - Water (as required)

Benefits:

- Rich in L-ascorbic acid - Bolsters resistive framework - Facilitates absorption - Provides hydration

Storage:

Refrigerate in an airtight receptacle for a maximum of 2 days. Vigorously shake before serving.

HARMONIZED FRUITS 4

PINEAPPLE HEAVEN FUSION

Preparation:

1. Sliceand corea fresh pineapple.

2. Dice the pineapple into chunks.

3. Introduce the pineapple chunks intoa blender and puree.

4. Puree until smooth.

Ingredients:

- Fresh pineapple

- Water (if necessary)

Benefits:

- Bromelain is present toaid digestion - Abounds in Vitamin C and manganese

- Boosts immune system - Possesses anti-inflammatory traits

Storage:

Refrigerate for up to 3 days in an airtight receptacle. Vigorously shake before serving.

HARMONIZED FRUITS 5

MELON MAGIC SYMPHONY

Preparation:

1. Handpick and slice your preferred melon (watermelon, cantaloupe, or honeydew).

2. Remove the seeds and rind.

3. Slice the melon flesh.

4. Introduce the melon chunks intoa blender and puree.

5. Puree until smooth.

Ingredients:

- Watermelon, cantaloupe, and honeydew

- Water (if necessary)

Benefits:

- Cooling and hydrating

- Rich in vitamins Aand C

- Promotes skin well-being - Facilitates digestion

Storage:

Refrigerate for up to 2 days in an airtight receptacle. Vigorously shake before serving.

HARMONIZED FRUITS 6

TROPICAL BREEZES FUSION

Preparation:

1. Strip and dice ripe bananas.

2. Shed and slice the skin off fresh papaya.

3. In a blender, merge banana slices and papaya chunks.

4. Blend until velvety.

5. For added creaminess, infusea splash of coconut milk.

Ingredients:

- Ripe bananas - Fresh papaya - Optional coconut milk

- Water (if needed)

Benefits:

- Abundant in vitamins Aand C - Facilitates digestion - Provides vigor - Contains digestiveenzymes

Storage:

Indulge in an impregnable vessel for a maximum of 48 hours. Vigorously shake before serving.

HARMONIZED FRUITS 7

APPLEORCHARD SYMPHONY

Preparation:

1. Strip, core, and slice theapples.

2. Position theapple pieces in a blender.

3. Blend until velvety.

4. Optionally, season with a hint of cinnamon.

Ingredients:

- Apples - Optional cinnamon

- Water (if needed)

Benefits:

- Bursting with fiber

- Bolsters heart health - Assists in weight reduction

- Maintains blood glucose levels

Storage:

Indulge in an impregnable vessel for a maximum of 48 hours. Vigorously shake before serving.

HARMONIZED FRUITS 8

KIWI KALEIDOSCOPE REFRESHER

Preparation:

1. Strip and thinly slice the kiwi fruit.

2. Clean and slice the kale leaves.

3. In a blender, merge kiwi slices and kale leaves.

4. Blend until velvety.

5. If desired, add a dash of lime juice.

Ingredients:

- The kiwi fruit

- Kale leaves (optional) - Lime juice

- Water (if needed)

Benefits:

- Abundant in vitamin C and K - Overflowing with antioxidants - Facilitates detoxification - Enhances the immune system

Storage:

Indulge in an impregnable vessel for a maximum of 48 hours. Vigorously shake before serving.

HARMONIZED FRUITS 9

SUNSET PEACH SOOTHER

Preparation:

1. Rinseand peel ripe peaches, then extract the pit.

2. Strip and cut the peach flesh into bits.

3. Position the peach chunks in a blender.

4. Blend until velvety.

5. Optionally, drizzle with honey for sweetness.

Ingredients:

- Ripe peaches

- Optional: honey

- Water (if needed)

Benefits:

- Abundant in vitamins Aand C - Enhances skin health - Facilitates digestion - Hydrates

Storage:

Indulge in an impregnable vessel for a maximum of 48 hours. Vigorously shake before serving.

HARMONIZED FRUITS 10

GUAVA GLOW ELIXIR

Preparation:

1. Clean and peel the guava fruit.

2. Extract the seeds from the guavaand cut it into bits.

3. Position the guava chunks in a blender.

4. Blend until velvety.

5. Optionally, squeeze in some lemon juice.

Ingredients:

- The guava fruit

- Optional: lemon juice

- Water (if needed)

Benefits:

- Abundant in vitamin C

- Boosts the immune system

- Facilitates digestion

- Enhances skin health

Storage:

Indulge in an impregnable vessel for a maximum of 48 hours. Vigorously shake before serving.

Conclusion:

Remember that the advantages listed are just a glimpse of what each juice has to offer. These recipes provide a splendid chance to personalize to your liking, experiment with diverse combinations, and relish the health benefits of a symphony of harmonizing flavors.